The Shocking Truth about Male Hair Loss

Secrets You Need to Know About Losing Hair So You Can Stop From Going Bald.

James Dobovin

Introduction:

I first started losing my hair when I was about 45 years old.

Of course, I panicked and started trying to cover the remaining hair with strange hairstyles that made me look silly in strong wind.

In compiling my hair information books my goal was to amass both informative and useful information.

Entwined in my words are long scientific words that are necessary if you decide to do further research. If they bother you just skip over them.

Along the way I found it difficult to locate facts about hair loss that was understandable and centrally located. Not wishing others to have such a difficult time I decided to put them all in one place. My individual hair information books include Male Hair Loss, Female Hair Loss, Saving Your Hair and Hair Diseases.

I sincerely hope that you learn some useful facts that will help you in your quest to save your hair.

Thanks and make it a healthy hair day.

James Dobovin

Disclaimer

Please note: This book is only for information purposes. This book is not intended to be medical advice and it is not a substitute for professional medical advice. Please consult your doctor for your medical concerns. Please follow any tips given in this article only after consulting your doctor. The author is not liable for any outcome or damage resulting from information obtained from this book.

Cure your Baldness & Alopecia the Natural Way (Chinese Herbs)

A recent media broadcast on UK television as part of an experiment to cure alopecia and treat thinning hair and baldness discovered the beneficial factors of using Chinese herbs in treating alopecia.

There are a number of Chinese herbs that can be beneficial for this condition. Chinese medicine treats the root imbalances in the body that result in alopecia. When the body is brought into balance, symptoms resolve themselves and slowly disappear.

The first is a pattern of Liver and Kidney Deficiency. This means that the energy of the body that normally nourishes the hair follicles is deficient. When herbs are used to nourish the Liver and Kidney, hair can start to grow back.

The second pattern is toxic heat in the body. This means that there is an inflammatory condition in the body that is a result of excess acidity from a poor diet, exposure to pollution or other toxins, or an infection. In most people with alopecia areata, these two conditions exist in combination with each other.

It is necessary to reduce inflammation and acidity in the body while nourishing the cooling yin energy of the body that nourishes hair growth.

Fo-ti has been used traditionally in China for graying hair and premature hair loss. It is a general tonic for the brain and the body, and can improve the quality of hair growth on the head. It can take three to six months of use to see the full benefits of Fo-ti. The Chinese have also traditionally used this herb as a longevity tonic.

Ligustrum and eclipta are two other Chinese herbs used to nourish hair growth by strengthening the liver and kidney Yin energy of the body. Research done in China has shown that these herbs can promote hair growth in people with alopecia areata.

Chinese wolfberries are also a general body tonic that improves blood circulation to hair follicles of the head. This herb can work well in combination with the herbs listed above.

In order to clear the inflammation and acidity that can trigger alopecia, mint, dandelion, and honeysuckle herbs can be used in combination.
Some supplements that may be of benefit in combination with Chinese herbs include vitamin C, flaxseed oil, and nettle tea.

All of these are anti-inflammatory and detoxifying to the body. Eating black beans and black sesame seeds can also be helpful when taken alongside Chinese herbs.

Chinese herbs are a safe, natural, effective, health-promoting way to treat alopecia areata and increase hair growth.

Encourage Healthy Hair with Hair Care Tips

Hair is an important aspect of an individual's appearance. It is natural and is determined at the time of birth. It generates from the number of roots in the scalp. Each hair grows up to a certain length and then stops naturally. It even sheds down at some point. New hair shaft replaces the lost hair. This new hair needs to be taken care of.

Healthy hair is a mirror to a good health. But due to the velocity of life one tends to skip over health issues leaving apart hair care. Here are a few hair care tips to ease hair loss and achieve manageable healthy hair.

Balanced Diet: Hair being a part of your body is affected by the food intake of an individual. It is recommended that a daily diet should be balanced with adequate amount of carbohydrates, fats, vitamins, proteins and minerals. An individual having oily hair should avoid intake of oily food items. Drinking plenty of water cleanses the toxins in turn enabling healthy hair growth.

Natural Hair Care: Brushing your hair regularly to stimulate the scalp will keep it looking healthy and lustrous. Never attack wet hair with a brush, no matter how rushed for time you are. Tangles in wet hair are best removed with a wide-toothed comb. A warm oil scalp massage two or three times a week will help stimulate and moisturize the scalp.

Air dry: Blow drying your hair robs off the excess moisture. It damages your hair even more. Let your hair air-dry whenever possible. Stand under the fan and run your fingers gently through the hair helping it dry.

Various hair care products are available in the market to help your hair restore its natural health and protect it from chemicals. Hair gels, creams, oils, shampoo, conditioner and hair softeners are to name a few. A wide range of hair care accessories in hair spray, tweezers, hair scissors, hair cutting scissors, sheers, professional sheers, hair sheers, hair comb, bobby pin, head band, eyelash curler, hair brush, and shower cap accessories are available.

For each hair care accessory and product, a full description of the product, picture of the package and the directions for its use is given.

In order to purchase a hair care product or accessory, one need not go searching for a salon or beauty shop. You can order it online. It's the easiest way to purchase the right product to spruce your hair.

Healthy hair is a blessing. Treat your hair right for lustrous and healthy hair.

Falling Hair? Cure It with Simple Scalp Exercise

A receding hairline is the most obvious sign of aging, being on the most prominent location. It is like falling leaves when autumn comes.

Caring for your hair doesn't stop with washing and shampooing it. You have to pay equal attention to it in the same manner as you pay to other parts of your body. The hair needs nourishment just like the rest of your system to keep them in place and keep them from moving to your bathroom shower drain.

In your campaign for a healthier body most of the time the hair is not included. You work out every inch of your body, but not the hair. There are no exercises for it anyway, you might think. But decades ago, Sanford Bennett, became a celebrity for experiments that led to his physical rejuvenation at 70. Besides all the exercises he devised to make his face younger and his bodily muscles more robust, he also devised an exercise for a healthier and stronger scalp that could trigger the thicker growth of the hair.

To Bennett, the scalp, just like any other part of the body if exercised, would increase in strength and elasticity. This is because there are microscopic glands and muscles in the scalp. The law that applies in exercising the major muscles of the body also applies to those.

So how does it go? Alternately pull your hair in all directions and massage the scalp with the pads of your fingers while you lie in bed. This will improve the blood circulation and eventually feed the roots of the hair with the nutrients it needed. It also exercises the muscles in the scalp making the muscles stronger, which will logically hold the hair more strongly.

And since the blood is pumped through the microscopic glands and muscles in the scalp, they are sure to increase in size, strength and elasticity. This naturally results in much fewer hair falling and healthier-looking hair.

One of the best refreshers for the hair ad the scalp is the alternate washing of hot and cold water. It also accelerates the blood circulation there. Wash the hair first with hot water, as hot as you can bear it.

Then follow up with very cold water (but without using ice). Applying hot and cold towels alternately can be a good substitute. This procedure should be repeated at least five or six times.

About Hair Loss

Any hair loss in excess of 10% of all hair at any point of time can be called abnormal hair loss and may require treatment or special care. Hair loss can occur on account of any of the following:

• Side Effects of medication
• Abnormal hormone levels
• Infection of the scalp
• Physical uprooting of hair because of poor head gear or bands
• Genetic reasons

The hair loss on account of any specific reason like medication, abnormal hormone levels or infection of scalp can be treated. The most troublesome and the most common forms of baldness is the common male/female baldness in which the hair recedes along the temples and the forehead in case of men and recedes in density all over in case of women. Such baldness is usually genetic.

Genetic baldness is usually caused by an enzyme alpha reductase that converts testosterone to dehydrotestosterone (DHT). DHT leads to shrinking of hair follicles. This results in generation of thinner and weaker strands of hair that fall off very quickly.

The special herbal hair care product Renew contains a group of herbs that provide overall scalp and hair root nutrition and also help in the control of dandruff. The special herbs in Renew help in stopping hair follicle shrinkage. Regular use leads to reversal of shrinkage and hair gain. Renew is helpful in all kinds of hair loss situations.

Renew is available in the form a hair oil that has to be applied locally. Local application means that unlike when systemic hair loss medicines like Fenasteride and Dutasteride, hair growth does not happen in undesirable areas like the back.

Massaging of hair and scalp with Renew provides additional nutrition to the scalp and prevents hair loss. Massaging also increases the blood circulation in the scalp and this keeps the hair roots strong.

Part your hair and apply Renew all over the scalp, massage the scalp gently with fingers in a circular motion so that the oil gets absorbed into the scalp. Leave for an hour and then wash with mild shampoo if required.

Alternatively you could apply Renew to your hair and scalp before going to sleep and then wash your hair in the morning.
Renew has no known side effects.

Each 10 ml of Renew oil contains:

Eclipta Alba 3%
Herpestis/Bacopa Monnieria 2%
Emblica officinalis 2%
Cyperus scariosus 1%
Vetiveria zizanioides 1%
Santalum album 1%
Pongamia glabra 1%
Crataeva nurvala 0.5%
Abrus precatorius 0.5%
Glycyrrhiza glabra 0.5%
Nardostachys jatamansi 0.5%
Valeriana jatamansi 0.5%

Andropause and Hair Loss

Andropause and hair loss often go hand in hand. Imagine clumps of hair falling off your head, or observing strands of once healthy hair collecting in the shower drain. Maybe you run your hand through your hair and feel it thinning. It can feel daunting and quite scary.

Typically, hair loss is a result of an imbalance of male testosterone hormone in the body. Instead of infusing the hair with healthy testosterone, enzymes break it down to a simpler form known as dihydrotestosterone.

An excess of this hormone has the effect of decreasing the size of hair follicles which eventually break down and make your hair fall off sporadically.

The medical condition that is best associated with hair loss in Andropause sufferers is hyperthyroidism. Hyperthyroidism is a by-product of decreasing levels of Human Growth Hormone, which is responsible for regulating our aging process.

Andropause sufferers' hormones have a profound effect on the rate and consistency of hair loss. Dihydrotestosterone (considered by medical circles the strongest, most potent form of testosterone) is responsible for building and growing body hair in men (at normal levels - an excess causes hair degeneration.)

This includes body hair, pubic hair, head hair, armpit hair – any hair. DHT is directly produced in the skin, made to work by supporting enzymes that break it down for distribution throughout the body. DHT levels are present more in certain areas of the body than in others – explaining why we may have a full crop of hair on our heads and little bushes of hair on our chests and backs.

Realize, women also have DHT in their bodies but produce less of it.

That explains why women don't have body hair. Case in point: an excess of DHT is prevalent in Andropause sufferers, explaining the reason for hair loss. The enzyme used to break down testosterone to dihydrotestosterone is "over activated" - working too hard and too fast.

This is the primary cause for this Andropausal condition. As aforementioned, dihydrotestosterone is present more in certain areas of the body than in others. For this reason, men's hair can fall into funny patterns. The shrinking of hair follicles as a result of the production of DHT is attributed to this.

How hair grows is a wondrous thing in itself that needs to be recognized. Typically, hair grows at a rate of a quarter inch every 2 weeks. Andropause sufferers have their "hair growth cycles" disrupted when there is erratic growth of some hair strands where "new" hair pushed "old" hair out.

Because Andropause is a period of hormonal imbalance, a lack of hormonal stability and poor homeostasis (holistic balance) in the body pushes things out of whack.

If you want to maintain healthy strands of hair, one thing you can do is hit that stair climber machine. Exercise reverses the aging process and may certainly reverse this symptom. There are also hair loss products that can help you recapture your hair.

Secondary causes of hair loss in men suffering Andropause is stress. More specifically, stress raises the levels of cortisol and cortisone (known as stress hormones) in the body. Eating non-nutritional foods also speeds up hair loss.

Pretty much any activity that speeds up the aging process will speed up your hair loss.

Stay away from caffeinated drinks, fast foods, and cigarette smoking to keep running your hands through your thick mane longer. Participate in recreational activities to reduce stress and light up your life with a proper exercise regimen.

If you're suffering from this condition, don't let it affect you in the least bit! Andropause should not serve as a punishment – rather, a realization of a future for the better.

The information in this article is for educational purposes only, and is not intended as medical advice.

Balding Solution for Men and Women

Androgenetic alopecia (male and female pattern balding) is by far the most common cause of hair loss amongst men and a serious problem for many women.

There are three important components which are responsible for both female and male balding:

1. A genetic predisposition for balding to occur.

2. Excessive presence of male hormones.

3. Aging - enough time for the first two factors to occur.

Both men and women produce male hormones that have a useful role to play in both sexes; but the fact that androgens occur in much higher concentrations in men explains why male pattern baldness is more common than the female balding.

DHT is the root cause of hair loss.

It is metabolism of male hormones (androgen/testosterone) which is main cause of hair loss and male and female pattern balding both in men and women.

The metabolism of androgen involves an enzyme called 5 alpha reductase which combines with the hormone (testosterone) and converts it to DHT (Dihydro-testosterone). DHT is a natural metabolite of our body.

Some individuals, both men and women, are genetically pre-disposed to produce more DHT than the normal individuals. It is this accumulation of DHT and its effect on the cells inside the hair follicle and root which is one of the primary causes of male and female pattern balding.

When DHT gets into the hair follicle and root, especially a region called the dermal papilla, it changes the cell' activity and prevents necessary proteins, vitamins and minerals from providing nourishment needed to sustain life in the hairs of those follicles.

Consequently, hair follicles are reproduced at a much slower rate. This shortens their growing stage (anagen phase) and or lengthens their resting stage (telogen phase) of the follicle. DHT also causes hair follicle to shrink and get progressively smaller and finer.

This process is known as miniaturization and causes the hair to ultimately fall. DHT induced androgenetic aloepcia is responsible for 95% of all hair loss.

Blocking the synthesis of DHT at the molecular level forms the basis for the treatment of MPHL (male pattern hair loss) and FPHL (female pattern hair loss). There are many natural DHT blockers and a number of drugs which are used for medical hair restoration.

Biotin and Hair Loss

The article 'Biotin and Hair Loss' emphasizes on root cause of hair problems i.e. Biotin deficiency in the body. After reading this article you will be aware about hair problems and will be able to solve them with the help of experts. You will also become aware about properties of Biotin, a vitamin of B complex group sometime also known as vitamin H or vitamin B7.

Falling hair is normal, when you take bath roll in the bed, do combing and such other activities, you lost some of your hairs. It is very natural. But if your hair falls and that too in such a quantity that makes your head poor haired then it is a deficiency, which may ultimately lead to baldness.

If this is the case, then you are suffering with hair problems. The causes may be many and you need to identify them, but ultimately your body is deficient of Biotin. Yes, Biotin, it is the vitamin, which makes your hair healthy, strong and good looking.

It is clinically proven, so maintaining a good level of Biotin in your body system is as essential as maintaining other vitamins and minerals. Biotin is necessary for your hairs health and overall well being. Medical specialists advise that the persons suffering with Hair Problems must take Biotin in addition to other medications.

So if you are suffering with hair problems, must go for medications with Biotin substitutes. Foods like egg yolks and liver contain a lot of Biotin, you need to consume these foods in rich quantity to maintain your health and prevent hair loss.

Using a Biotin enriched shampoo may also help in improving your hair health.

Some more foods rich in Biotin are; brewer's yeast, green peas, oats, soybeans, walnuts, sunflower seeds, green peas, bulgur and brown rice, etc. Eating these foods and food products will help your body in maintaining a good level of Biotin.

A person who is a patient of heartburn, acid reflux or GERD absorbs less amount of Biotin, and hence may trap into hair problems. This is because; a person suffering with above-mentioned disease takes a lot of antacids.

So now, you will definitely agree with the fact that Biotin is a hair food, and important for good hair health.

What else does Biotin do for your body?

Biotin is a member of Vitamin B complex family also sometime known as Vitamin H or Vitamin B7. This is soluble in water, which means, if body has high level of Vitamin H at a certain day or time, it pass out through Urine. This vitamin is produced in the intestine with the help of bacteria in the intestine.

Biotin helps in metabolism of carbohydrates, fats and proteins and helps in maintaining steady blood sugar. So, it is good for the persons suffering with Diabetes. Diabetes is a major disease across the globe and affects several men and women.

Biotin does process glucose and we know glucose is one of the source of energy of our body to perform work and maintaining wear and tear of the body. Biotin also helps in making of DNA, RNA and nucleic acids and production of fatty acids. Growth and replication of cells depends on Biotin.

Thus on one hand Biotin helps in maintaining good hair health and on the other hand it is important for several bodily functions.

Sources of Biotin:

The main sources of Biotin are; liver, kidneys, milk, cheese, butter and other dairy products, egg yolks, oysters, lobsters, poultry, cauliflower, avocados, bananas, strawberries, watermelon, grapefruits, raisins, mushrooms, green peas, blackcurrants, brewer's yeast, wheat germ, nuts, beans, lentils, oat bran, whole grains, oatmeal, peanut butter, molasses, and foods like salmon, tuna, mackerel, and herrings (foods rich in Omega – 3 fatty acids).

A healthy person and pregnant woman must take 300 grams of Biotin in daily diet. Breastfeeding mothers need about 350 micrograms of Biotin.

Symptoms of Biotin Deficiency

People affecting with Biotin deficiency may show dry or scaly scalp, a loss of appetite, hair problems; closely associated with Biotin deficiency, nausea, depression, dermatitis, anorexia, and anemia.

Can Too Little Protein Cause Hair Loss?

Hair usually grows about half an inch per month, although this slows as you age. Each hair remains on your head for two to six years, and during most of this time is continually growing.

But many factors can disrupt this cycle. The result can be that your hair falls out early or isn't replaced.

A new discovery has been made in finding out what actually causes hair loss, namely: the hardening of collagen. Persons who do not suffer from hair loss have ample collagen.

But many factors can disrupt this cycle. The result can be that your hair falls out early or isn't replaced.

A new discovery has been made in finding out what actually causes hair loss, namely: the hardening of collagen. Persons who do not suffer from hair loss have supple collagen and persons who begin showing signs of hair loss have hardened collagen.

Collagen hardening interferes with the healthy functioning of the hair roots. The vital exchange process of the hair follicle cycle is disrupted and the hair becomes suffocated.

But What Causes Hair Loss?

Diet: Too little protein in your diet can lead to hair shedding. So can too little iron. Bottom line: Too strenuous dieting can result in hair loss! If you want to lose weight, do it the sensible way, especially if you have a hair thinning/loss problem to begin with.

Childbirth: Some women lose large amounts of hair within two to three months after delivery.

Hot Tips!

One great tip is after washing your hair, dry it in whatever manner you normally do. Then turn your head upside down, give your head a vigorous shake, and once back in a standing position, either "place" your hair using your fingers, rather than a brush or comb.

You can also use a hair pick to style your hair. The upside down, shaking, also gives a great deal of fullness to otherwise flat looking thin hair. You'd be amazed at how creative you can be with your fingers without pulling at the root of the hair!

To protect hair, the best practice is to shampoo only when hair is dirty. Because fine hair gets dirty faster, people with fine-textured hair need to shampoo more frequently -- even though fine hair breaks more easily.

For that reason, fine-textured hair benefits from a good shampoo and volume-building conditioner

Hair Diseases Resulting in Hair Loss

It is sometimes found that a particular hair loss cause is more commonly related to a particular hair disease. In this context one can refer to the acquired hair shaft defects. These defects are usually triggered by the excessive use of hair treatments and styling products.

Hair diseases and hair loss are interrelated. One cannot be thought about without the other.

Common hair loss causes

No single factor can be marked out as the universal cause of hair diseases. There are several causes varying from person to person.

The two types of hair loss diseases:

The hair loss causes can be broadly divided into the following two groups

The temporary effect and the one involving a prolonged action, usually triggered by genetics.

a.) The temporary effect – Usually such cases can be cured by medications and treatments.
b.) Prolonged hair loss diseases – Such cases may require long term treatment. Sometimes the drug treatment might appear to be ineffective. In such circumstances surgery like hair transplantation may be the way.

The causes of temporary hair loss include the ones like child birth, using birth control pills, etc.

Another key factor can be hormonal imbalance. It can have a severe impact by causing pattern baldness. The latter comes in the list of major hair diseases.

Relation between hair diseases and hair loss:

It is sometimes found that a particular hair loss cause is more commonly related to a particular hair disease. In this context one can refer to the acquired hair shaft defects. These defects are usually triggered by the excessive use of hair treatments and styling products.

Similarly, infectious diseases have their root in unhygienic scalp.

The common causes of hair loss diseases include the following –

- Hormonal imbalance
- Ailment
- Faulty hair styling
- Inadequate diet

Hormonal Imbalance

In men – Hormonal imbalance is a major cause of hair loss diseases among men. The male hormone testosterone plays a key role in actuating hair loss. The enzyme 5 alpha reductase in the hair follicles turns testosterone into dihydrotestosterone (DHT). The latter is the most potent androgen promoting male pattern baldness, the common hair loss disease.

In women – Imbalance in thyroid hormone is a key cause of sudden hair loss among women. The thyroid gland's being n the state of overactive and under active might cause hair fall. Thyroid hormones largely influence cellular metabolism of scalp proteins, carbohydrates, lipids and minerals. And the hair matrix cells are highly affected by the thyroid hormones' excess or deficiency.

Hormonal imbalance also causes hair loss during pregnancy. Pregnancy witnesses a high level of estrogen hormones. This causes hair follicles percentage in anagen growth phase. But post-child birth there is a rapid fall in the estrogen level. Consequently a large number of hair follicles shift to a catagen phase. And gradually hair falls.
Women may also experience hair loss during post-pregnancy period. It is generally temporary in nature. But if it continues for months, then it may indicate hormonal imbalance in the body. And hormonal imbalance for an extended period requires proper treatment.

Ailment

Some of the serious ailments like high fever, severe infection, or flu may lead hair follicles to a resting phase. This condition called telogen effluvium results increased hair fall. But it is a temporary condition soon to be followed by normalcy.

Some cancer treatments also prevent the hair fiber growth. The hair becomes thin and breaks off. And gradually hair loss occurs. The condition starts within one to three weeks after the beginning of the chemotherapy treatment. The treatment may witness the patients losing up to 90 percent of their scalp hair.

Faulty hair styling

It means using certain hair styling techniques resulting in hair loss diseases like traction alopecia. In this condition the hair fibers are pulled out from the hair follicle by a hairstyle that pulls on the roots of the hair fibers. One example of such faulty hair styling is braiding corn rowing.

Cosmetic treatments like bleaching, coloring or hair straightening like chemical relaxing can also create problems if proper procedure is not followed.

Inadequate diet

Taking up crash diets for rapid weight loss may lead to hair loss. Such diets are low in protein, vitamins and minerals, thus causing malnutrition. Abnormal eating habits lacking important nutrients can also result into hair loss.

Hair Loss: Don't Rule Out a Thyroid Condition

If you suffer from hair loss you might want to make sure that your problem is not caused by a thyroid condition.

Although the usual reasons for hair loss are genetic predetermination, hormonal changes, or certain cancer treatments, thyroid hair loss should also be considered.

There are three types of hair loss;

Thyroid hair loss, autoimmune alopecia, and male pattern hair loss.

Thyroid hair loss can manifest in both hyperthyroidism and hypothyroidism. In those with thyroid hair loss, there will be a general thinning of the hair, without the bald patches characteristic of male pattern baldness.

Symptoms of hypothyroidism include fatigue, dry skin, abnormal sensitivity to cold, constipation and depression. If you one or more of these symptoms along with loss of hair, think about getting tested for thyroid problems.

Synthroid is commonly prescribed in hypothyroidism; this medication is effective however, it can produce thyroid hair loss as a side effect for some people. Your hair loss may be due to Synthroid, so speak to your doctor about the possibility.

Thyroid hair loss can also occur if you are under-treated. A Thyroid Stimulating Hormone level of around 1-2 is optimal for a large number of people who are suffering from hypothyroidism with no hair falling.

Evening primrose oil supplements are one alternative therapy that some have found to be useful in alleviating thyroid hair loss. Aromatherapy is another which is reported to be effective.

Essential oils of thyme, cedar wood oil, lavender, and rosemary can be blended and applied to the scalp to help encourage hair growth.

Ayurveda medicines such as Bhingaraj oil or brahmi oil have also been used to treat hair loss due to thyroid conditions. Both these oils applied to the scalp continuously for at least 3 months are said to aid hair growth. Growth of hair will also be aided by supplementation with the ayurvedic herbs amla and ashwagandha.

The ultimate remedy for thyroid hair loss is hair transplantation. Tiny hair plugs are removed from the scalp's back or side and then implanted to bald portions of the scalp. Results can be seen after several months. This procedure is expensive and is not always covered by insurance providers, but can be worth every penny for those suffering from this discouraging condition.

Hair Loss: Aloe Vera Treatment and Other Natural Hair Loss Treatments

Many people feel that the problem of hair loss cannot be solved with the help of hair loss treatment products. They often get frustrated after spending too much money on ineffective hair loss remedies and their side effects with no positive results at all.

In reality, hair loss treatment can be divided in two categories: Natural hair loss treatments and chemical treatments.

Here are some best hair natural hair loss treatments:

Aloe Vera

Indians, Native Americans and Caribbeans have used Aloe Vera to promote healthy hair and prevent hair loss since ages. Aloe Vera balances the pH of the scalp and heals from within. It is also helpful in cleansing the pores.

A general remedy of Aloe Vera gel with coconut milk and small amount of wheat germ oil used as a shampoo has shown great benefits. Aloe Vera surely helps you stop hair loss.

Jojoba

If you are affected with hair problems like eczema, psoriasis, dandruff or seborrhea you are requested to use jojoba oil. Native Americans and Mexicans have used jojoba oil for centuries to prevent hair loss and to control dandruff. Jojoba oil works well for hypoallergenic skin, as is a good moisturizer. This is one of the best hair loss treatment products.

Henna

Henna is a traditional Indian herb, which is a good natural conditioner and works great as hair loss treatment product. It heals hair shaft by sealing the cuticle and repairing, stops breakage and restores the silky-shiny effect of your hair.

Capsicum

It stimulates hair growth by 50% and increases flow of blood to the scalp. This herb is effective in preventing hair loss.

Lemongrass

This herb helps stabilizing oil product in the scalp. It also provides nourishment to the hair. You can use oil of lemongrass for massage as well.

Dong Quai

Formation of DHT is the main cause of hair loss. Dong Quai contains phytoestrogens, which reduces the formation of DHT. Hence, Dong Quai is believed to be helpful in hair loss.

It is recommended that you consult an expert to know which hair loss treatment product is suitable for you.

The Top 3 Reasons for Losing Your Hair

According to scientists, there are three causes of alopecia in either men or women.

Too much DHT
Pseudo-estrogen chemicals
Lack of vital nutrients

DHT

Free testosterone is broken down into DHT (a more potent form of testosterone). This chemical binds to the hair follicle receptors blocking vital nutrients from accessing the hair.

The hair becomes miniaturized and thin and eventually dies. It is what's called the "peach fuzz" look on young men with hair loss.

This is why eunuchs never had any hair loss which got Plato wondering. It is also why only men get male pattern baldness and women don't. Hair loss in women is more evenly distributed with a thinning over the whole scalp.

Also, effective DHT inhibiting treatment was only effective on young men with hair loss and not older men or women. Excessive DHT is therefore not the only reason for losing your hair.

Pseudo-estrogen Chemicals

It is normally unheard of for women in China to get hair loss at any age. Over the last 20 years increasing number of Chinese women in the industrialized areas of China are experiencing hair losses.

This has been put down to chemicals form the industrial process which mimic the chemical effects of estrogen.

These pseudo-estrogen chemicals bind tighter to the hair follicle receptors than normal estrogen does, starving the hair follicle of vital nutrients, similar to the way DHT does.

Also, this seems to the reason for hair loss in obese men. Fat cells in obese and balding men contain more of the enzyme aromatase (responsible for converting testosterone into oestrogen). Also bacteria in fat cells produce oestrogen-like chemicals.

Lack of Vital Nutrients

The hair needs a variety of nutrients to sustain it. The theory is that both DHT and estrogen-like chemicals block the hair follicle by binding to it too tightly. Even without these chemicals, a person lacking in these nutrients will experience hair loss.

There have been experiments on mice which show the effect of a deficiency of certain vitamins or minerals. Scientists knocked out the genes in mice responsible for the regulation of the hair and scalp.

These genes are in turn normally regulated by vitamin D.

The result was rickets and hair loss with dermal cysts appearing quite early on. When scientists injected naturally "nude" mice with vitamin D, they started sprouting hair at an alarming rate.

It has been shown that copper and zinc, if lacking together, increase a loss of hair. In fact, a copper peptide was shown to induce hair growth in the skin around the wound of a person. The copper peptide was first used as healing accelerant.

For women, a lack of iron and the essential amino acid L-lysine has been associated with losing one's hair. This therapy has proven to be very beneficial for women who are losing their hair.